How to lose weight as a teenager

The secrets to maintain an ideal weight as a teenager

Ben Williams

ISBN9781724143730:

[ii]

PREFACE

These book will be discussing extensively on losing weight of teenagers starting from the foundation of teenagers (Adolescent) to important and vital nutrients intake important for every teens. Parents role in educating teenagers about how to stay healthy. Being of healthy weight allows for proper metabolism of the body and able to carry out our day to day activities.

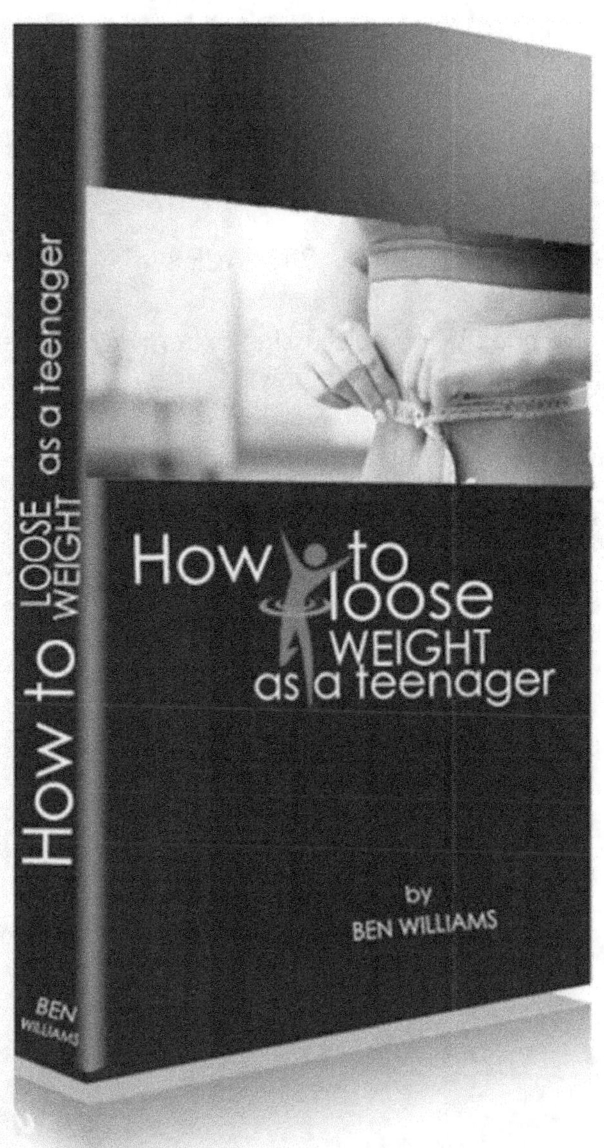

How to loose WEIGHT as a teenager
by
BEN WILLIAMS
How to LOOSE WEIGHT as a teenager
BEN WILLIAMS

TABLE OF CONTENTS

PREFACE

TABLE OF CONTENTS

CHAPTER ONE

CHAPTER TWO

CHAPTER THREE

CHAPTER FOUR

CHAPTER FIVE

CHAPTER SIX

CHAPTER SEVEN

Ben Williams

HOW TO LOOSE
WEIGHT AS A TEENAGER

BEN WILLIAMS

CHAPTER ONE
INTRODUCTION

A teenager, or teen, is a person who falls within the ages of thirteen-nineteen years old. A teenager is another word for an adolescent. When a teenager turns 20, they are no longer a teenager because they are no longer in that developmental stage. Adolescence is the name for this transition period from childhood to adulthood. In the United States, children and teens from the ages 11–14 go to middle school, while teenagers from the ages of 14–18 typically go to high school. In the United Kingdom, teenagers and children are mixed in secondary school. Teenagers attending secondary school (high school in the US) generally graduate at the age of 16 or 19.

An adolescent is someone going through puberty. A teenager is someone in the age of 13 to 19. Therefore they don't have to be going through puberty at that time, since the beginning of puberty varies for different people. It could start at 14 or even 11 (dependent on gender). Therefore they are two separate categories, they just seem similar.

1.1 MEANING O.F ADOLESCENCE

Adolescence means 'to emerge' to achieve 'identity' not only in physical or intellectual aspects but also in his/her whole human hood, which includes emotional or psychological, social and spiritual. The time of growing up from childhood to adulthood is known as the

Adolescence. It is a period of physical growth; a time for the maturing of mind and behaviors as well. The length of time for this period of development varies. Adolescence can start at nine (9) and end at eighteen (18). It can start at fourteen (14) and end at twenty five (25). Young people may grow quickly in some ways and more slowly in others. This is why children who may be only 9, 10 or 11 years old may be Adolescents in some ways already, while teenagers of 13 or 14 may just be reaching Adolescence. On the one hand reaching out towards adult roles and on the other still needing the love and protection of parents. It is a time when children undergo a crisis of identity.

The term "Adolescence" comes from the Latin word 'adolescere' that means "to grow" or "to grow to maturity". Maturing involves not only physical but also mental growth. It is a period, which fills the gap between childhood and adulthood. Generally, this period is termed as "youth". According to A.T. Jersild, "Adolescence is a span of fears during which boys and girls move from childhood to adulthood mentally, emotionally, socially and physically". In India Adolescence is a phase that is more difficult to define, particularly in terms of age. The classic age-wise grouping for Adolescence is between 11 to 18 years for girls and between 12 to 18 years for boys. .Dorothy Rogers has viewed this period as a process of achieving the attitudes and belief needed for effective participation in the society. Thus, there is no absolute age limit for a clear-cut boundary between the Adolescence and adulthood. Adolescence is the stage between childhood and adulthood. It is not an age, but a stage. In India, the Adolescent is a person who has not been sufficiently recognized and encouraged. Due to financial reasons the Adolescent is dependent on his parents for many more years than in the West. The emotional dependence is also as great, producing what is termed 'Delayed Adolescence'. Adolescence is between 12 to 20 years. A delayed Adolescence goes on until 21 years and even up to 25 years.

1.2 STAGES OF ADOLESCENCE FORMATION

1. Early Adolescence: Early adolescence is from 10 to 12years. The rate of growth increases, starting first in the hands and feet and later in the limbs. In early Adolescence, they start initiating independence from the family, and desire for privacy. There may be a clash between the wish for their autonomy and parental authority.

2. Middle Adolescence: Is from 12 to 16 years. The peak of the height velocity curve is seen auxiliary hair and sweat glands develop. In 80% of girls the dramatic event of menarche occurs. The timing for this is influenced by genetic factors and nutritional status. Any chronic illness can delay puberty. The eruption of the second permanent molar and menarche closely correspond in timing. In middle Adolescence, the school and peer group gain importance. Girls develop into personal skills quicker, loyalty and commitment matter more, shared information becomes important. Decisions of vocations and education are made. Physical maturation can influence school performance and

aspirations for better achievement because the physical effect of pubertal development becomes incorporated into the self-image. These is the stage for TEENS AND TEENAGERS

3. Late Adolescence: Is from 16 to 19 years. The body approximates the young adult and development of secondary sex characteristics is completed. In late Adolescence, career decisions are finally traced. The child gradually returns to the family, on a new footing.

1.3 DEFINING ADOLESCENCE ACCORDING TO CATEGORIES

- CHRONOLOGICALLY, Adolescence ranges from age 12 to 18 years.
- LEGALLY A boy who is of the age between 12-18years would be termed as minor or juvenile (Adolescent) who also means to say that he has not attained his maturity. Whereas in the case of girls the age group of 12 – 21 years would be termed as minor or juvenile (Adolescent). Legally Adolescence ends with the assumption of adult responsibility for voting.
- SOCIOLOGICALLY it is a period, which fills the gap between dependent childhoods to self-sufficient adulthood. In addition, they are generally termed as youth and characterized as hot-blooded in nature. 10Socially it ends with marriage.
- MEDICALLY adolescence begins with the growth and a hormonal change associated with sexual maturity and ends when there is no further growth. The adolescent period between puberty and the completion of physical

growth is roughly from 11 to 19 years of age. The period of adolescent development is between the onset of puberty and adulthood. This period is generally marked by the appearance of secondary sex characteristics, usually from 11 to 13 years of age, and spans the teen years.

• EDUCATIONALLY adolescence is the time spent in high schools and early

colleges.

• PSYCHOLOGICALLY it is a period of transition, during which cognitive,

physical, personality and social changes occur.

W.H.O defines adolescence both in terms of age spanning the ages between 10 and 19 Years.

1.4 GROWTH AND PHYSICAL DEVELOPMENT OF TEENAGERS

The phenomenal growth that occurs during teenagers is second only to the growth that occurs during the first year of life, and it increases the body's demand for energy and nutrients. Nutri- tion needs are greater during teens than at any other time in the life cycle. During this period, teenagers achieve the final 15 to 20 percent of their adult height, gain 50 percent of their adult body weight, and accumulate up to 40 percent of their adult skeletal mass. Nutrient needs parallel the rate of growth, with the greatest demands occurring during the peak period of growth (sexual maturity rating [SMR] 2 to 3 in females and 3 to 4 in males). For females, most physical growth is completed by about 2 years after menarche. (The mean age of menarche is 12 1/2 years.) Males begin puberty about 2 years later than females, and they typically experience their major growth spurt and increase in muscle mass.The changes associated with puberty affect ado- lescents' satisfaction with their appearance. For males, the increased size and muscular development that come with physical maturation usually improve their body image. However, physical matu- ration among females may lead to dissatisfaction with their bodies, which may result in weight con- cerns and dieting.

Nutrition and physical activity are major determinants of teens energy levels and influence growth and body composition. Inadequate nutri- tion can delay sexual maturation, slow or stop lin- ear growth, and compromise peak bone mass. Practicing healthy eating behaviors and participat- ing in regular physical activity can help teenagers achieve normal body weight and body composition, thereby reducing their risk of obesity.

1.5 THE BODY WEIGHT

Body's relative mass or the quantity of matter contained by it, giving rise to a downward force; the heaviness of a person or thing.Human body weight refers to a person's mass or weight measured in kilograms or pounds in some other regions in the world. Body weight is very vital in accessing and monitoring body fat or muscle mass changes, or for monitoring hydration level.To get reliability of body weight, weigh routinely in the morning (12 hours since eating). Body weight can be affected by fluid in the bladder (weigh after voiding the bladder). Other conditions are:

1.   the amount of food recently eaten,

2.   hydration level,

3.   the amount of waste recently expelled from the body,

4.   recent exercise and clothing.

In cases of changes in body weight which you are not such of, reweigh at the same time of day, under the same conditions with no clothes / shoes on. These will be give optimum result if otherwise compare using another measuring scale. guidelines for proper and efficient determination of body weight is standing with minimal movement with hands by their side. Shoes and excess clothing are not allowed.

1.5.1   Calculating your body weight

A highly physical teen boy with great muscle tone could easily weigh higher than average on the standard average height and weight chart. This is due largely to the fact that muscle cells weigh more than fat cells. Due to this, a more common measure of average healthy bodies is based on a formula known as the Body Mass Index or BMI . To determine how much you should weigh (your ideal body weight) several factors should be considered, including age, muscle-fat ratio, height, sex, and bone density. Some health professionals suggest that calculating your Body Mass Index (BMI) is the best way to decide whether your body weight is ideal. Others say that BMI is inaccurate as it does not account for muscle mass, and that waist-hip ratio is a better method. BMI uses weight and height to determine whether an adult is within the healthy weight range, underweight, overweight or obese .It provides an estimate of total body fat and your risk of developing weight-related diseases.Your BMI is a measure of your weight in relation to your height

It's worth remembering that one person's ideal body weight may be completely different to another's. If you compare yourself to family and friends you risk either aiming too high (if you are surrounded by obese or overweight people), or too low (if everyone around you works as a fashion model). Even comparing yourself with people outside your immediate surroundings may not work. BMI is a very simple measurement which does not take into account the person's waist, chest or hip measurements.

BMI is calculated by dividing weight by the square of height as follows:

BMI = Weight (kg)/Height (m)

Use the health direct BMI calculator to work out your BMI. The calculator indicates any health risks in relation to your BMI or waist circumference, and offers information based on your personal results. To calculate your BMI yourself, it is important to make sure you measure your weight in kilograms and your height in centimeters. To find your weight classification (if you are an adult), see which of these BMI ranges your weight falls into:

Under 18.5 Underweight (In some countries health authorities say the lower limit for BMI is 20, anything below it is underweight).

18.5–24.9 Healthy weight range / ideal

25.0–29.9 Overweight

30.0–34.9 Obesity I

35.0–39.9 Obesity II

40.0 (and above) Obesity III

1.5.2   Limitations of BMI

1.   BMI is less accurate for assessing healthy weight in some groups of people because it does not distinguish between the proportion of weight due to fat or muscle. BMI is therefore less accurate in certain groups, including:

- certain ethnic groups among the Chinese and Japanese population groups
- body builders or weight lifters
- some high-performance athletes
- pregnant women
- the elderly
- people with a physical disability
- people with eating disorders
- people under 18 years
- those with extreme obesity

2.   Experts say that BMI underestimates the amount of body fat in overweight/obese people and overestimates it in lean or muscular people.

CHAPTER TWO
IMPORTANT NUTRIENTS

Not all teenagers may have the same nutritional requirements. Nutritional needs may also vary by gender. Maintaining your body weight been a teenager requires proper nutrition and lifestyles, Healthy eating is providing the right balance of nutrients the body needs each and every day. These specific nutrients the body requires as a teenager are to be provided in a balanced diet daily:

1. Calcium rich food; Proper calcium levels are important for developing strong bones. More than one-third of your adult bone mass is deposited during teenagers. Inadequate calcium intake put teens and teenagers at risk for developing osteoporosis later in life. The recommended amount of calcium is 1,200 mg every day. Low fat dairy products (such as milk and yogurt) are good choices to make up the difference. So it is advisable to replace your soft drinks with milk. Since milk contains fortified vitamin D, it also helps in strengthening the bones

2. Iron; Iron is an important mineral as it facilitates the

delivery of oxygen to the tissues and develops the brain and immune function. Iron also provides the body adequate energy to function. Boys and girls need adequate amounts of iron to support their rapid growth. During growth spurts, iron helps new muscle cells obtain oxygen for energy. The recommended amount of iron for girls is 15 mg per day and for boys is 12 mg per day (girls need a little more iron to account for menstrual losses).

Iron deficiency causes anaemia leading to fatigue, weakness and decreased learning ability. Other good sources of iron include lean meats, fortified whole grain cereals, spinach, fish and shellfish.

3.   Protein; protein is important for growth, energy and the repair of body tissues (muscles). Protein is very satisfying/filling macronutrient that it helps to curb hunger easily.Teenagers require protein for proper growth and development being a building block for muscles, bones, skin, blood, hormones and enzymes. All teenage girls needs 5oz proportion of protein each day. Teenage boys who are 13 needs 5oz of protein a day, and teenage boys older than 13 needs 6 ½ oz equivalents. An ounce equivalent of protein may consist of 1 egg, 1 tbsp. of peanut butter, one-half-oz. serving of nuts or seed or a 1 oz. serving of poultry, fish or meat.

4.   Fluids: water is the best fluid; so ensure to drink the recommended 6 to 8 glasses of water in a day so that you don't feel dehydrated. You can include other fluids like unsweetened fruit juices and milk.

5. Fruits and Vegetables: Fruits and vegetables are an excellent source of vitamins and minerals needed by a growing teen body. So it is advisable to consume five servings of fruits and vegetables every day. These can be easily taken in the form of baked or steamed veggies, fruit juices and smoothies. You can also try fresh, frozen or dried fruits as optional snacks.

Vegetables also contain numerous vitamins and minerals without providing unnecessary calories, sodium or fat. Vegetables are also a good source of dietary fiber. Teenage girls who are 13 years old should get 2 servings of vegetables, and female teenagers older than 13 should get 2 ½ cups of vegetables a day. Teenage boys who are 13 years old should get 2 ½ servings of vegetables, and teenage boys older than 13 should get 3 cups of vegetables a day. A serving of vegetables can be a 1 cup of vegetable juice, 1 cup of raw or cooked vegetables or 2 cups of raw leafy greens.

Fruits provide numerous vitamins and minerals, including nutrients that many teenagers don't get enough of such as fiber, vitamin C, folate and potassium, according to the USDA. Teenage girls between the ages of 13 and 18 should get 1 ½ cups of fruit a day, and 19-year-old females should get 2 cups of fruit a day. Teenage boys who are 13-years-old should get 1 ½ cups of fruit, but all other teenage boys should get 2 cups of fruit a day. A cup of fruit may consist of 1 cup of fruit juice, one-half cup serving of dried fruit or 1 cup of raw or cooked fruit.

6. High Fiber Foods: Foods that are high in fiber can keep you full for longer, thus keeping hunger at bay and minimizing calorie consumption. Sources of fiber include whole breads, whole grain cereals and fruits and vegetables.Grain products are a good source of dietary fiber, B vitamins, iron, magnesium and selenium. The daily grain recommendations for teens are based on ounce equivalents. An ounce equivalent may include a 1/2 cup serving of cooked rice or pasta, 1 cup of cereal or one slice of bread. Thirteen year old girls should get 5 oz. of grain a day, and girls who are between the ages of 14 and 19 should get 6 oz. equivalents of grain a day. Thirteen year old boys should get 6 oz. of grain a day, and boys between the ages of 14 and 19 should get 9 oz. equivalents of grain a day. All teens should aim to get at least half of their grains from whole grain products.

7. Diary: since bone mass is built during adolescence, diary intake during the teenage years is especially important. All teenagers, regardless of age or gender, should get 3 cups of dairy each day. A cup of dairy is equal to 1 ½ oz. of natural cheese, 2 oz. of processed cheese, 1 cup of yogurt, 1 cup of soy milk or 1 cup of milk.

8. Supplements from food sources: Most teenagers can meet their nutritional needs through a balanced and healthy diet, but taking a multivitamin can help ensure that the recommended dietary allowance of each vitamin and mineral is met

2.1 STAGES OF NUTRIENTS INTAKE

Nutritents are taken in proportion and stages of the day including breakfast, lunch and supper. The importances of each meal are stated below

1. Usefulness of Breakfast

Breakfast is the most important meal of the day aiding in memory and concentration at school, and energy supply during study and play.Teenagers having regular breakfast tend to have a healthier weight than those who skip breakfast. Breakfast meals should be high fibre and low fat and with not too much added sugar or salt. Here are some healthy breakfast options:

1.1.1.   porridge with honey and cinnamon

1.1.2.   muesli with yoghurt

1.1.3.   fresh fruit and yoghurt

1.1.4.   higher-fibre cereals like wild oats

1.1.5.   multigrain toast with a boiled or poached egg

1.1.6.   baked beans on toast

1.1.7.   raisin toast

1.1.8.   pita bread with olives and feta

1.1.9.   melted cheese and vegemite on toast or an English muffin

1.1.10. crumpets with jam

1.1.11. banana milkshake or fruit smoothie

1.1.12. pancakes with yoghurt and fruit.

2.   Usefulness of lunch

Lunch are exciting meals because they are lightweight which does not have to be boring, it must be compelling and admirable. Below are suggestions:

1.1.1. Chicken, grated carrot, cucumber and cream cheese pita bread

1.1.2. Turkey, cheese and salad on multigrain bread

with cranberry sauce

1.1.3. Vegetable and lentil soup in a thermos with a bread roll

1.1.4. Smoked salmon, salad and cream cheese bagel

1.1.5. Leftover pasta with lots of cooked vegetables

1.1.6. Quiche and salad

1.1.7. Cheese and salad sandwich

1.1.8. Boiled egg and salad on multigrain with a smear of mayonnaise

1.1.9. Ham, cheese and spinach wrap

1.1.10. Cold cooked cheese, salad and lean meat quesadillas

1.1.11. Chicken with avocado and salad in a grainy bread roll

1.1.12. Beef, tomato and lettuce sandwich with tomato chutney or salsa

3   Eating for study

While at school or studying, the brain needs extra energy. Eating healthy foods is also linked to better concentration. The following are tips for eating healthier when studying and during exams.

1.1.1. Eat small frequent meals.

1.1.2. Easy and convenient nutritious meals include: frozen dinners, tinned soups, peanut-butter sandwiches, breakfast cereal, cheese sandwiches, tuna or chicken and salad sandwiches, baked beans or eggs on toast.

1.1.3. Snack foods like chips and lollies can cause you to feel grumpy, irritable and low in energy. That's not what you want while you are studying. Try healthier snacks such as yoghurt, nuts, dried fruit, fresh fruit, plain popcorn or vegie sticks with dip.

1.1.4. People use caffeine for a 'pick me up' to feel more awake or alert. Too much caffeine from coffee, tea, cola and energy drinks can disrupt your sleeping patterns, send your heart racing, make it difficult to focus and/or cause nervousness in some people. Try sticking to one or two cups of coffee or tea a day, or try decaffeinated coffee or herbal teas as an alternative. Enjoy cola or energy drinks only occasionally as they have too much sugar and little nutritional benefit.

1.1.5. Drink plenty of water. When you are dehydrated you can feel tired.

1.1.6. Eat only when you are hungry. Be aware of your hunger signals, like stomach pangs, grumbling guts, dry mouth etc. If you need a study break and do not have hunger pangs, have a drink of water or go for a walk.

1.1.7. Regular exercise helps to improve your blood circulation, which keeps oxygen and nutrients flowing to your body and brain helping you to concentrate.

4   Eating for sport and play

Eating good foods before exercise can boost stamina and endurance. The following will help:

1.1.1. breakfast cereal with milk and fruit

1.1.2. dried fruit and nuts

1.1.3. yoghurt and fruit

1.1.4. English muffin with peanut butter and honey

1.1.5. banana and peanut-butter sandwich

1.1.6. fresh fruit smoothie with milk and/or yoghurt

1.1.7. low-fat muesli bar

1.1.8. small muffins made with oats or wholemeal flour and fruit or vegetables

1.1.9. low-fat custard and fruit

1.1.10. raisin toast and cream cheese

1.1.11. sushi handrolls

1.1.12. fruit scone

1.1.13. trail mix with dried fruit, nuts, seeds and some choc chips

CHAPTER THREE
ACHIEVING A HEALTHY WEIGHT

It is very convenient and comfortable as teens and teenagers to grab sweet foods like biscuits, potato chips, cakes, sausage rolls, pies, doughnuts or chocolate bars when you are hungry, but it poses a risk regularly choosing these foods because they add more calories which will make it easier to put on more weight. Its of utmost importance to enjoy these kinds of convenience food (takeaway and fried foods) occasionally only. Other things to avoid are drinks with lots of sugar, for example, fruit juice, cordial, soft drinks and energy drinks.

Sugar is of 2 types;

i)   Simple sugar

ii) Complex sugar

The simple sugar is glucose, fructose while the complex sugar are cellulose, glycogen and starch which are then broken down into the simple sugars. Most of the food and drinks we take in have sugars but drinks from fruits blended naturally with no other agents are the best in achieving and maintaining our weight unlike drinks with lots of sugar which adds up to our calories. Every food we take in must be balanced in nutrients and calories.

The following table are breakdown of various drinks with its size and amount of sugar always added to it during production.

250 ml drink	No of teaspoon sugar
Coke cola	3
Low fat milk	3
Diluted cordial	4 ½
sports drink	3 ½
Energy drink	5
Orange juice	4
Iced Tea	4

1 teaspoon equals 5g of sugar

Here are some healthier alternatives to your usual snack foods or fast-food.

Don't take these	Take these
Chocolate bar 50 g	Low-fat chocolate milk drink 250 ml
Lollies	Dried fruit
Large coffee	Small coffee
Ice-cream	Low-fat frozen yoghurt or sorbet
High-sugar breakfast cereal	High-fibre cereal e.g. untoasted muesli
Hot chips	Baked potato
Large soft drinks	Small soft drinks, diet soft drink or water mixed with lemon or lime.
Fried egg and bacon	Poached egg and ham in an English muffin

3.1   HOW TO KNOW IF I AM OF A HEALTHY WEIGHT

As a teenager, the body is through a stage of growth and development. Its normal to add more weight as the bones and muscles develop likewise the body structure. At times you possess enormous strength to do anything and some other times you don't. Ideally if you eat healthy in the form of a balanced and well proportioned meal you will be amazed to know how your appetite is guided by the number of calories and nutrients for growth and development for your day to day activities. However in cases of too much eating of food, overweight is achieved. Being overweight is a dangerous problem than just the way you look or feel leading to serious health problems like diabetes, high blood pressure, lung disease or heart disease in adult life. Similarly not having regular meals has its own problems from affecting energy levels, growth and development. Loss of vital nutrients such as calcium.

CHAPTER FOUR

EFFICIENT AND EFFECTIVE TIPS TO MAKE YOUR TEEN EAT HEALTHY

These are guidelines to parents or guardians, teens are often under guidance and protection of parents and guardians. As a parent or guardians, here are a few easy and effective tips on how to promote healthy eating habits for teens:

1. Persuade, coerce them and not force teens about eating healthy: One of the first things you need to do is remember your teens about the importance of healthy eating, don't in any way try to push or force the issue Talking about eating healthy and eating together can inspire your teen to eat better. Instead of making it a daily debate topic, talk to your teen about it at regular breaks. Make sure you do not sound preachy or angry. Do not make it sound like a power issue but something like a heart to heart chat between a parent and a teen. Encourage your teen to eat healthy by providing a variety of healthy eating options at home. Show your teen that healthy does not have to mean boring and bland. Try out new recipes as and when you can.

2. Get Your Teen Involved: Your teen will be more fulfilling and easier to connect to healthier food if she is involved in the food which can be done by giving him/her the responsibility of planning one meal a day. Ask her to try and include as many healthy options in the meal as she can. Set her a challenge of coming up with delicious and interesting food ideas by giving her a pre-set selection of ingredients and putting a timer. Make it a game rather than a rule. Shop together with your teen at local farmers' market and encourage her to pick the items himself.

3.   Make Them Informed: Teen's and teenagers blindly follow junk food habits as a result of peer pressure.it's your job to make your teen understand the negative effects of settling in for junk or food items that are not healthy. Share news articles and health videos that show the real face of unhealthy foods. Let your teen see why foods from popular food chains are termed unhealthy.

Teach your teen how to read labels and then find out how many unhealthy ingredients are there in his favorite ready to eat snack. Encourage your teen to research and come up with information himself.

4.   Stock Your Home With Healthy Eating Choices: In most cases, your teen will easily reach out for foods that she can see in his line of vision. Make sure you fill up your home with healthy eating options like fruits, fresh vegetables, healthy herbs and spices and more. Keep fruits and some raw vegetables like tomatoes, carrots and more, in a small basket on the table where your teen can get them easily. .Instead of stocking up on packaged juices and such, prepare fresh juice right in the morning and keep it on the family table. You can also keep jars of fruit infused water on the table that your teen can sip on through the day.

5. Lead By Example: Your teen may not admit it, but in most cases, what you do will greatly impact your teen's overall behavior. Make your food selections wisely and incorporate healthy eating habits before expecting the same from your teen. If you or your partner suffer from any health issues, tell your teen about it and discuss what eating habits could have prevented it.

CHAPTER FIVE

LOSING WEIGHT AS A TEENAGERS

Losing weight as a teenager is all about lifestyle management and not dieting. Lifestyle management by a teenager includes the following:

### 1.	Avoid Skipping Meals:

Skipping meals is actually counter-productive when it comes to losing weight. In fact, you should eat frequent small portions every 3 to 4 hours in a day. You should try and consume at least five meals a day. Eating several small portions will also keep your blood sugar level steady. Most people have this misconception that skipping breakfast is a great way to cut calories. But the fact is, when you skip breakfast, you experience hunger pangs and end up binging during lunch. Certain studies have also observed that people who eat breakfast tend to have lower BMIs.

### 2.	Drink Plenty Of Fluids:

Drinking fluids does not mean you have to gorge on aerated drinks, sodas and processed juices as they load your body with calories. Water is the best liquid that not only hydrates your body but also removes toxins from your system. It is advisable to drink at least 3 liters of water in a day. Other fluids you can consume include unsweetened fruits juices diluted with water and low fat milk. Green tea is also a great option to lose weight. Fruit and vegetable juices are devoid of fiber, so eating whole fruits and vegetables is a better option.

3.   Replace Your Chewing Gum With Mint:

Teenagers are often habituated to chewing gum. It does help in burning calories but is not good for your stomach. Chewing causes you to swallow more puff-producing air instead of food. You can try sucking a mint instead of chewing gum. Besides keeping hunger at bay, a mint will also give you fresh breath.

4.   Don't Eat Anything After 8 P.M:

Late night snacking is certainly not conducive to weight loss. So it is advisable to finish your dinner by 8 p.m. You can indulge in a cup of tea or frozen yoghurt if you need something sweet after dinner. But late night munching should be avoided as much as possible as whatever you eat gets stored in the body as fat. Brush your teeth after dinner to ensure that you do not indulge in snacking between 9 p.m. to 6 a.m.

5.   Give Up Unhealthy Snacks And Processed Foods:

Most of us love to snack on chips, French fries, cakes, sausages, biscuits, pies and candies. However delicious they may be, they are high in unhealthy saturated fats and sugars that can lead to weight gain. These food items also lead to high cholesterol. To become fit, these should be replaced with healthier options like fruits and vegetables. Now these might not look like an attractive alternative but these can be made interesting. You can have them with peanut butter or hummus. You can also munch on a handful of unsalted nuts or popcorn without added salt or butter. Greek yoghurt also helps boost your metabolism and can be eaten topped with honey and berries.

6.   Stay Away From Fat:

Fat foods are a big no; especially if you wish to lose weight on a long term basis. Numerous fad diets promise quick weight loss and they do yield results. But these results are short lived and are often accompanied by nutritional deficiencies and health risks. As a teenager, you require adequate supply of all vital nutrients to fulfill your body's growth requirements. Fad diets are nutritionally unbalanced and so the weight lost in the course of diet is likely to be regained after the diet is over. So it is important to choose your diet plan carefully to incorporate a healthy balanced diet with more physical activity.

7.   Do Not Follow Low Carb Diets:

Several low carb diets are gaining prominence these days. But they can prove to be unhealthy as they often eliminate whole food groups, thus depriving you of the nutrients from those food groups. These diets are often high in saturated unhealthy fats that can cause high cholesterol and increase the risk of heart disease. Some other diets eliminate dairy foods like milk, yoghurt and cheese. These food items are a good source of calcium which is vital for healthy bones and their proper growth. So think hard before you decide to get on a diet.

8.   Exercise Regularly:

To be able to lose weight successfully, you need to make exercising a part of your daily routine. Physical activity is important for the fitness of both body and mind. You can lift weights, swim or run on a treadmill. You can perform simple exercises like squats, dips and crunches at home. Even dancing is a great exercise that works on all your body muscles. Ensure to exercise at least 3 to 4 days in a week rather than being a couch potato.

9.   Walk As Much As You Can:

Walking is also a great way to burn calories. An average person can burn 6 calories by walking for a minute. Begin by walking one mile a day and remember to walk at a brisk pace. Slow down if you find yourself out of breath and increase the distance to be covered gradually. Use the stairs instead of lift. According to certain studies, walking for 15 minutes in a day can increase your life expectancy by 3 years. This is one of the easy ways to lose weight for teenagers

10.　Read food labels.

When you read a food label, pay special attention to:
• Serving Size. Check the amount of food in a serving. Do you eat more or less? The "servings per container" line tells you the number of servings in the food package.

•Calories and Other Nutrients. Remember, the number of calories and other listed nutrients are for one serving only. Food packages often contain more than one serving.

•Percent Daily Value. Look at how much of the recommended daily amount of a nutrient (% DV) is in one serving of food—5-percent DV or less is low and 20-percent DV or more is high. For example, if your breakfast cereal has 25- percent DV for iron, it is high in iron.

11.　Turn off the TV and get moving!

Can too much TV contribute to weight problems? Several research studies say yes. In fact, one study noted that boys and girls who watched the most TV had more body fat than those who watched TV less than 2 hours a day. Try to cut back on your TV, com- puter, and video game time and get moving instead. Here are some tips to help you break the TV habit.
•Tape your favorite shows and watch them later. This

cuts down on TV time because you plan to watch specific shows instead of zoning out and flipping through the channels indefinitely.

• Replace after-school TV watch- ing and video game use with physical activities. Get involved with activities at your school or in your community.

12. Making It Work

Look for chances to move more and eat better at home, at school, and in the community. It is not easy to maintain a healthy weight in today's environment. Fast food restaurants on every corner, vending machines at schools, and not enough safe places for physical activity can make it difficult to eat healthfully and be active. Busy schedules may also keep families from fixing and eating dinners together.

13. Build muscle

Muscle burns more calories than fat. So adding strength training to your exercise routine can help you reach your weight loss goals as well as give you a toned bod. And weights are not the only way to go: Try resistance bands, pilates , or push-ups to get strong. A good, well-balanced fitness routine includes aerobic workouts, strength training, and flexibility exercises.

14. Forgive yourself

So you were going to have one cracker with spray cheese on it and the next thing you know the can's pumping air and the box is empty? Drink some water, brush your teeth, and move on. Everyone who's ever tried to lose weight has found it challenging. When you slip up, the best idea is to get right back on track and don't look back.

15. Schedule regular meals and snacks.

You can better manage your hunger when you have a predictable meal schedule. Skipping meals may lead to overeating at the next meal. Adding 1 or 2 healthy snacks to your three squares can help curb hunger

CHAPTER SIX

UNDERSTANDING YOUR ENVIRONMENT

Understanding your home, school, and community is an important step in changing your eating and activity habits. Your answers to the questions on this checklist can help you identify barriers and ways to change your behavior to support your success.

• Home

1. Is the kitchen stocked with fruits, vegetables, low-fat or fat-free milk and milk products, whole-grain items, and other foods you need to eat healthy?

2. Can you get water and low-fat or fat-free milk instead of soda, sweetened tea, and sugary fruit drinks?

3. Do you pack healthy lunches to take to school?

4. Does your family eat dinner together a few times per week?

5. Do you have sports or exercise equipment at home, including balls, bikes, and jump ropes?

6. Do you limit the hours you spend watching TV or playing video or computer games?

• School

1. Does the cafeteria offer healthy foods such as salads and fruit?

2. Are there vending machines in school where you can buy snacks and drinks like baked chips, fig bars, and bottled water?

3. Do you take gym class on a regular basis?

4. Are there after-school sports or other physical activities available aside from gym class?

• Community

1. Are there bike paths, hiking trails, swimming pools, parks, or that offer open fields that are safe to use?

2. Are there grocery stores fruits, vegetables, and other healthy foods?

3. Is there a community center, church, or other place that offers classes such as dance, self-defense or other physical activities?

4. Do the streets have sidewalks so you can walk safely?

CHAPTER SEVEN

CONCLUSION

As a teenager you can lose weight as a result of understanding balanced diet, cuting off sugars and practicing more of taking a walk, engaging in physical activity. These are all changes that are effective slowly. These changes will be scary and not an easy task that's why you must set a few realistic goals for yourself. First, try cutting back the number of sweetened sodas you drink by replacing a couple of them with unsweetened beverages. Once you have reduced your sweetened soda intake, try eliminating these drinks from your diet. Then set a few more goals, like drinking low-fat or fat-free milk, eating more fruits, or getting more physical activity each day. Then identify your barriers. Are there unhealthy snack foods at home that are too tempting? Is the food at your cafeteria too high in fat and added sugars? Do you find it hard to resist drinking several sweetened so- das a day because your friends do it? Use the tips stated in these eBook to effect the change and complement your effort by

- Ask a friend, sibling, parent, or guardian to help you make changes and stick with your new habits.
- Know that you can do it! Use the information in this booklet and the resources listed at the end to help you.
- Stay positive and focused by remembering why you wanted to be health- ier—to look, feel, move, and learn better.

• Accept relapses if you fail at one of your nutrition or physical activity goals one day, do not give up. Just try again the next day.

Also, share this information with your family. They can support you in adopting healthier behaviors

AMAZING FACTS YOU NEED TO KNOW

• From 2003 to 2004, approximately 17.4 percent of U.S. teens between the ages of 12 and 19 were overweight.

• Overweight children and teens are at high risk for devel- oping serious diseases. Type 2 diabetes and heart disease were considered adult dis- eases, but they are now being reported in children and teens..

• Dieting is not the answer. The best way to lose weight is to eat healthfully and be physically active.

• A day keep you from putting weight, they'll help you feel full and keep your heart and the rest of your body healthy.

• Healthy weight and living requires long term success of forbidding sweet foods

• The brain needs 20 minutes to define you are full so therefore eating more slowly can help, taking a break before going for seconds can keep you from eating another serving

• Simply cutting out a can of soda or one sports drink can save you 150 calories or more each day.

• Small changes are a lot easier to stick with than drastic ones. For example, give up regular soda or reduce the size of the portions you eat. When you have that down, you can make other changes, like introducing healthier foods and exercise into your life.

• The best weight-management strategies are those that you can maintain for a lifetime. People who lose weight quickly by crash dieting or other extreme measures usually gain back all (and often more) of the pounds they lost because they haven't changed their habits in a healthy way that they can stick with.